Nitrogen Gas as an opportunistic poison; and

washout

therapies

drifting

in

the

fog.

Donald R VanDeripe

Dedication: To-

Deceased: Marjorie and Floyd (mom & dad), Gordon (brother), Judy (wife and mother of my daughters, Natalie & Nicole)

John and Dan (sons in law) and Alex, Nick, and Maggie (grandchildren),

and extended family.

Published: September 2015

Contact: Donald R. VanDeripe

P.O. Box 1637

O'Fallon, MO 63366

Foreword:

This will be my first and last book. Therefore I will include a brief autobiography to 'set the stage' prior to the scientific section. The science, if you will, is limited to basically four topics. <u>First</u>, there is a hypothesis and explanation of how the mitochondrial permeability transition pore acts as an oxygen pump to deliver oxygen into mitochondria for use in synthesis of adenosine triphosphate, and how this may be controlled by a biological feed-back system. Also, when oxygen becomes unavailable, the oxygen pump feedback system delivers nitrogen gas instead, thereby poisoning the mitochondria. The only chance to get rid of this this nitrogen is to wash out all of the nitrogen from the body and that can be accomplished by breathing heliox, a la deep sea diving. <u>Second,</u> there is discussion presented that, autism, Alzheimer's and other central nervous system diseases originate as impaired blood flow for several uncorrectable anatomical defects. However, their etiology and progression may, in part, result from elevated intracranial pressure (ICP). In the skull we have the brain, blood and cerebrospinal fluid (CSF) and the only way to decrease ICP is to remove fluid. Shunting of CSF to the peritoneal or pleural cavities has been successful, but is problematic. Decreasing the production of CSF through the use of carbonic anhydrase inhibitor drugs such as acetazolamide may effect a lowering of ICP with a resultant increase in cerebral blood flow. <u>Third,</u> the development of 'heliox' houses for chronic periodic nitrogen washout sessions is covered, but not in detail. The concept is simple. As nitrogen slowly fills brain mitochondria in chronic low blood flow diseases, daily, twice weekly, etc. washout sessions to salvage at-risk mitochondria might prove to be of value. <u>Fourth,</u> a mixture of the above and other topics.

Chapters: Page

CHAPTER 1 Autobiography

Why autobiography? I'm not writing about my car.

My name is Donald Ray VanDeripe (Don); I was born in 1934 in Lafayette, Indiana. For the first 6 +years we lived in Scircleville, Indiana (pop ~ 150), but moved back to Lafayette in '40 where my dad worked the night trick as a telegrapher for the Nickel Plate and Big Four Railroads during the war to keep the troop and supply trains moving. Here I must digress to cover my extreme talent in athletics. In neighborhood softball games I used to hit line drives to deep right field and get thrown out at first base. John Ave, a neighbor dad, said Donnie, you run harder than anyone, you just run too long in one place. When I went out for the track team in eighth grade, coach-Clark jibed- I'll have to retire my stop watch and by a calendar. Despite all this I played center on the Jefferson High freshman football team and we went nine and zero. However in my sophomore year things changed. I became drum major of the high school band and so we performed at halftime at the football games. This necessitated my dressing for football, then changing into the 'tall hat' outfit for halftime shows, then back again into football gear.

During pre-game warmup of our second home game (Kokomo), we were jogging out for passes to loosen up the QB, and it was my turn, so off I went, the QB dropped the ball, and what was to be a 15 yard toss became a 25 yard 'bomb'. Well, I jumped, it sailed over my head and I fell on my butt. The Kokomo fans howled. That made me realize that I should dump football and concentrate on music (I played clarinet and saxophone in the band). During high school and continuing through college I played in dance bands (Bob Doran, Carl Hedberg, and Wendy Schwartz); I enjoyed the latter the most, playing a baritone sax. The money from this helped with college expenses, but the most important help for college came after high school graduation in the form of a pivotal summer job.

My dad was friends with Charlie Sechrist (sp), foreman of a railroad section gang operating out of Lafayette, and they provided for me, a summer job as a section hand. Not wanting to embarrass my dad, I worked like a dog. Heat at 110F reflecting off the rails, number one at the bottom of transport car to heave 14 foot creosote covered switch ties up and out and drop them next to the track.

Then we had to slide these ties under two sets of tracks to secure them. Finally, for my last two weeks on the job, we were raising the tracks on the wide curve next to the Purdue Airport. This activity employed hand-held paddles powered by ~50 pound electric motor vibrators to shake the gravel and rocks under the ties. Each night after work and even at bedtime I had no feeling in my arms below the elbows, but all was well in the AM. When it was time to quit the job and start college, I had not embarrassed my dad since Charlie told him that I was the hardest worker on the crew that summer of '51. That experience not only convinced me to go to college but also, don't flunk out.

Selecting Purdue was easy since I lived only about 5 miles away and in-state tuition was low (would you believe $540.00 total for all four years?). I chose Pharmacy because of no foreign language requirement and only one year of math. Things went well and after 3 1/2 years I began to wonder where I might get a job. Dean Jenkins came to the rescue and addressed the class to the effect "we need graduate students". So I requested an interview. Therein, he indicated that I really didn't have the grades, but then noted that I had improved each year and he would give me a try. He asked which area I wished to pursue and I answered Pharmacology (it was my favorite subject). I indicated my postgraduate plan to the draft board. They laughed and said, go for it, you'll flunk out and we will see you in 6 months. Note: In 56-57, there was no active war conflicts, so the draft boards were lenient. The 12-14 months of grad school under the tutelage of C. Jelleff Carr and George KW Yim was quite enjoyable and resulted in a MS degree in Pharmacology. However, in those days there was an undertone circulating that advanced degrees in Pharmacology from Pharmacy schools were 'inferior' to those from Medical Schools. That was part of my decision to transfer to Northwestern University Medical School to pursue my PhD training. My faculty leaders there were Carl Dragstedt, Jay Wells and Julius B Kahn, the latter my major professor. [.......ASIDE: A Dragstedt definition: An expert is a former drip under pressure.......]. Well, starting in the fall of '58, I had to repeat all my course work, followed by two false starts on thesis projects. Finally I finished up in mid-63 and, thanks to Dr. Kahn, I moved on to a post-doc program in cardiovascular pharmacology at Emory U. under the direction of Dr. Neil Moran.

Time flew and I was soon interviewing for positions in academia or industry. I chose to go to Mallinckrodt in St. Louis and remained there for 30 years. We mainly did R&D on in vivo diagnostics (x-ray contrast media for Radiology and radiopharmaceuticals for Nuclear Medicine). First in Lab management, I moved into the administrative positions of technical evaluation and later the funding of outside research grants.

My own limited personal research carrier started in 1990 when I requested and received from my boss Ron Hopkins the opportunity to moonlight for one morning per week. That resulted in a research project which laid the groundwork for much that is contained in this book. The question I posed was- could gas and volatile anesthetics produce their pharmacological actions in the form of gas bubbles? My first efforts involved 5 rats, four of them anesthetized with methoxyflurane, halothane, ethyl ether and the gas nitrous oxide. The fifth rat served as an untreated decapitated control. All brains were harvested, dropped into 2% glutaraldehyde and processed for electron microscopy. All EM pictures showed gas bubbles, even the control rat. Sent off for publication, one reviewer commented: "the author has merely documented the presence of bubbles following the administration of anesthetics. No conclusions about mechanisms of action can be drawn for a descriptive study such as this." O.K., what is an editor's job? I would think it would be to identify new knowledge- –'merely documented the presence of bubbles'. Well Mr. Editor, the first report of gas bubbles in the brain (body) doesn't cut it? THAT caused me to shut down for a couple of years. Then I restarted with the agreement of boss #2 Leon Lyle. Several other anesthetics were studied in 26 additional rats and attempts to publish repeated with no takers. Finally in 1999, four years after retirement from Mallinckrodt, I met Dr. Steven Baskin, Editor of Toxicology Methods who personally helped me get published in that journal. Still, the article received scant, if any, attention because PubMed never picked up that journal for abstracting. Earlier this year however, the publisher, Taylor & Francis made the article available on-line.

CHAPTER 2: The Mitochondrial Permeability Transition Pore (mPTP).

What is the mPTP? It is a pump; more specifically, an oxygen pump. It pumps angstrom sized bubbles of oxygen from the cytosol through the outer mitochondrial membrane and transports them through the inner membrane into the mitochondrial matrix. There it becomes available for use in the synthesis of adenosine triphosphate (ATP). The presence of these oxygen bubbles is perhaps best demonstrated in a freeze-etched electron photomicrograph (EM) published by Hackenbrock [1], figure 1, page 5. The legend describes small particles confined to the molecular core of the outer membrane with larger particles confined to the inner membrane core. Hackenbrock does not specifically define the nature of the particles except to suggest that they are protein in nature. It appears to me that these structures are bubbles of oxygen coated with a very thin film of ice. Note: Hackenbrock states that the freeze-etched fixation occurs within one millisecond. The physical appearance of these 'bubbles' is that they are whitish or opalescent, not unlike refrigerator ice cubes. That is typical of ice cubes containing gas, not the clear ice cubes one gets from degassed ice machines. So, if the particles are ice coated gas bubbles, what gas? Physiology and biochemistry would certainly favor oxygen. How does this oxygen pump concept fit with current thought on the mPTP? It doesn't. Siemen [2] noted that more than 3434 publications on the mPTP were listed in Medline as of 2012. In his or any other of several reviews no one has associated failure of the mPTP to anything other than mitochondrial death and a resultant osmotic uptake of water which causes swelling of the mitochondria. Herein is provided evidence to support the author's hypothesis that mitochondrial swelling results from the mPTP pumping of nitrogen gas resultant from cytosolic hypoxia/anoxia. In 2001, the author reported on the mechanisms of action of gas and volatile anesthetics and obtained an EM of the brain from a decapitated control rat- PhotoEMA (page 6). Three giant mitochondria were observed all with transparent interiors (matrix). Number one showed three internal bubbles, number two a bubble in transport and all three showed a clear matrix with deformed and fragmented cristae pushed to the outer walls, indicating that the clear matrix (nitrogen gas) was immiscible with the cristae structures. A 75 second fixation delay of the rat brain would suggest that oxygen would be scarce (see chapter 3).

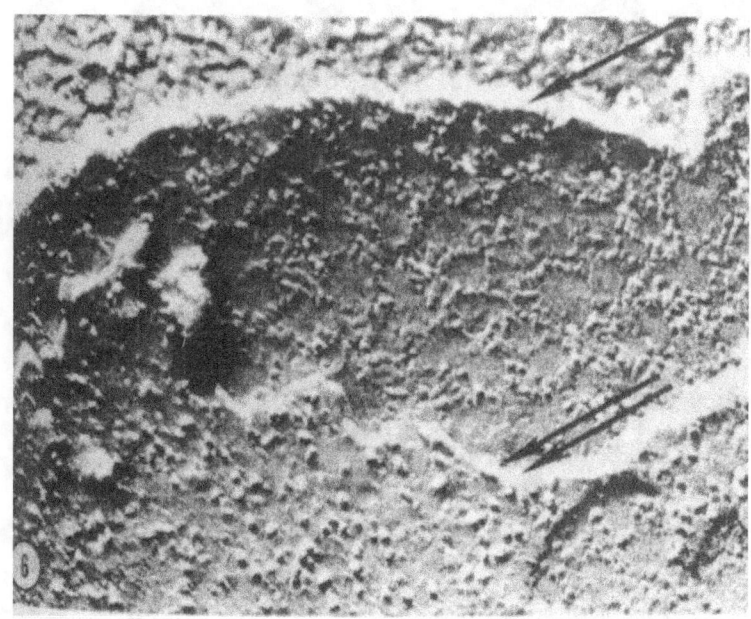

Figure 1. Electron microscope image of a mitochondrion from Hackenbrock [5]. "Concave fracture faces of the molecular core of the outer membrane (single arrow) and inner membranes (double arrow) of an energized orthodox mitochondrion. The inner membrane is torn away, exposing the fracture face of the molecular core of the outer membrane. The hexagonal arrays of small particles which surround smooth patches are seen to be confined to the molecular core of the outer membrane. The fewer, large particles, some randomly distributed and some in clusters and rows are confined to the molecular core of the inner membrane." Freeze-etched X137,500. Reproduced with permission of John Wiley and Sons, Inc.

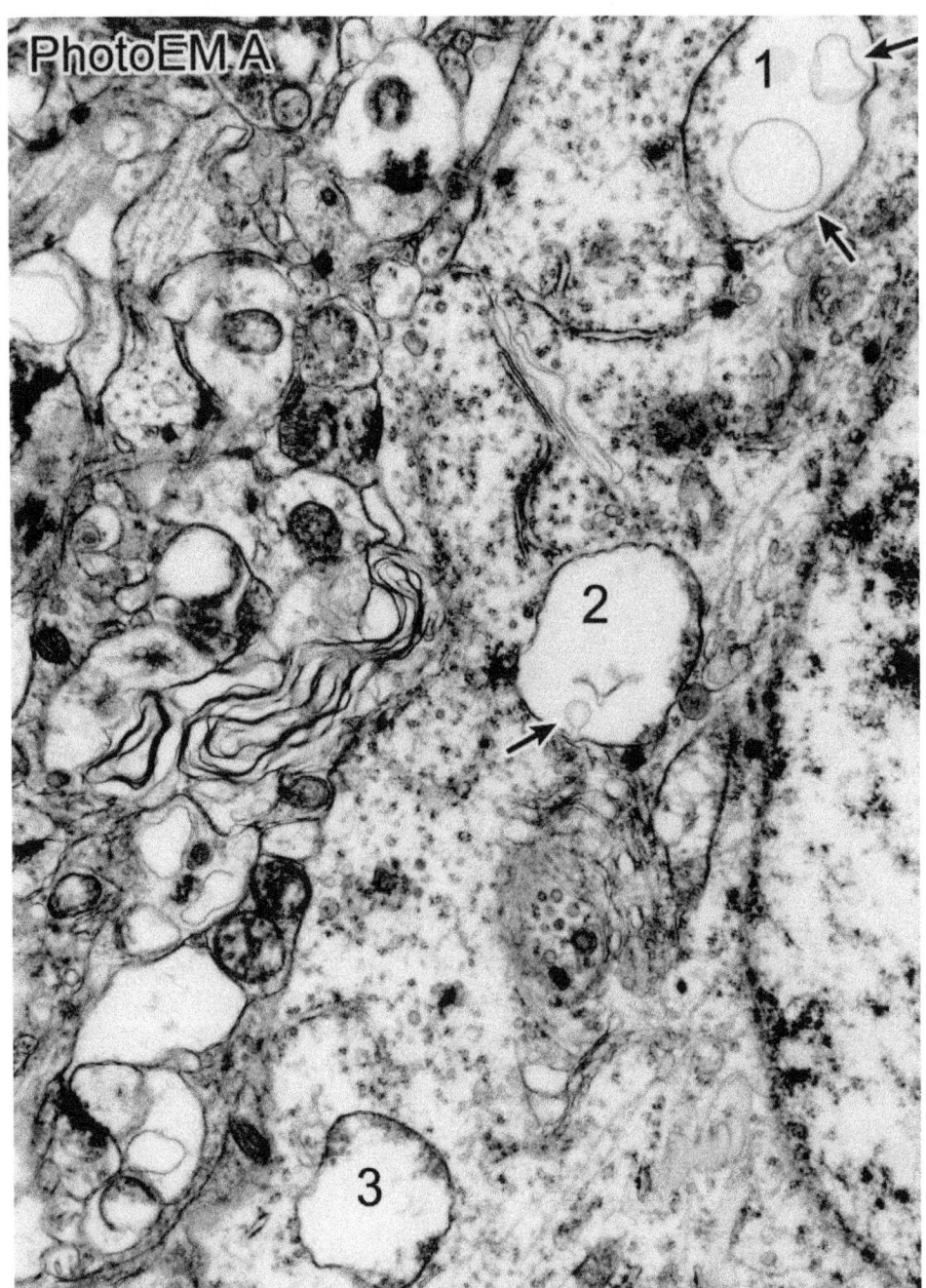

PhotoEMA: Control untreated rat brain gray matter X 24,900 fixed in 2% glutaraldehyde 75 seconds after sacrifice. Sample was post-fixed with 1% osmium tetroxide, embedded in Spurr's resin, sliced by ultramicrotome and viewed on a JEOL 100X transmission electron microscope. Three swollen (electron transparent) mitochondria demonstrate #1- interior gas bubbles, #2- gas bubble in transit into the internal matrix, and #s 1,2 and 3 deformed and fragmented cristae (periphery) not miscible with the nitrogen –swollen gas milieu. From Donald R. VanDeripe, Toxicology Methods 11; 107-126 (2001).   Copyright © 2001, Taylor&Francis Group, LLC; Informa Healthcare; PhotoEMA adapted with permission of Informa Healthcare.

Wakabayashi [4] describes mega-mitochondria as having diminished capacity to synthesize ATP. Kroemer notes that ATP and ADP inhibit the mPTP [5]. Siemen [2] is more specific indicating that the ATP inhibition is only from extramitochondrial (cytosolic) ATP. It is interesting to note in PhotoEMA, that the three massively swollen mitochondria are located perinuclear. If the nuclear membrane requires a higher turnover of ATP to maintain stability, that would fit with the observed mitochondrial swelling in this rat brain. This would also fit will with Siemen's comment that only external (cytosolic) ATP influences the mPTP. Taken together with Kroemer, these observations permit the following hypothesis of a feedback loop system.

[When cytosolic ATP and mitochondrial ADP levels are high, there is no need for additional oxygen and the mPTP oxygen pump rests and the mitochondrion assumes the condensed configuration. As cytosolic ATP levels drop the mPTP pump is signaled and pumps in oxygen leading to the orthodox (somewhat swollen) state. However, following a heart attack or stroke blood flow ceases and tissue hypoxia/anoxia develops. Then cytosolic ATP and/or internal ADP levels drop and the mPTP is signaled to pump oxygen, but, there being none available, pumps nitrogen gas instead. This signaling continues and the mPTP continues to pump nitrogen into the mitochondrial matrix even against concentration and pressure gradients to a point where massive swelling and membrane rupture can occur].

This all fits with the report of Leshnower [6] that cyclosporine inhibits the mPTP and in so doing blocks the mitochondrial swelling so often reported following myocardial ischemia/reperfusion studies in animals and humans (see chapter 3). All of this supports the authors contention that total body nitrogen washout by breathing heliox may be an effective therapy for mitigating reperfusion injury [7]. Moreover, it is the only approach that gets the 'toxic' nitrogen out of the body.

NEEDED EXPERIMENT: A definitive experiment to nail down this hypothesis would be to anesthetize a dog with pentobarbital and then immediately switch the respiratory gas mixture to heliox (30% oxygen/70%helium). Expirations would monitored for nitrogen content and then shunted to ambient air. Expired nitrogen levels should approach zero in about 40 minutes. After one hour, a coronary artery would be ligated for an hour, and then reversed to allow reperfusion for two hours. Then the dog would be sacrificed and a number of tissue samples obtained from normal and ischemic zones. These samples would be dropped into 2-3% glutaraldehyde and processed for electron microscopy. The data end point should be that the mitochondria in the ischemic zone should not be swollen at all or at a minimum and would be no different than those from normally perfused tissue. The absence of swollen mitochondria would provide a priori evidence that nitrogen gas is the causative agent for mitochondrial swelling, not water. In turn, such data would validate the hypothesis that the physiological function of the mPTP is to act as an oxygen pump in a feedback loop "system".

REFERENCES:

[1] Hackenbrock C.R. States of Activity and Structure in Mitochondrial Membranes. Annals New York Academy of Sciences 195; 492-505: (1972).

[2] Seimen D, Ziemer M. What is the Nature of the Mitochondrial Permeability Transition Pore *and What is it Not*? IUBMB Life. 65(3); 255-262 (2013).

[3] VanDeripe DR. Gas Microbubbles in Biology: Their Relevance in Histology, Toxicology, Physiology and Anesthesia. Toxicology Methods 11; 107-126: (2001).

[4] Wakabayashi T. Structural changes of mitochondria related to apoptosis: swelling and megamitochondria formation. Acta Biochim Pol. 46(2); 223-237: (1999).

[5] Kroemer G. Mitochondrial control of apoptosis: an overview. In-Mitochondria an Cell Death, Eds Brown C, Nicholls D, Cooper C. Princeton University Press, Princeton NJ pp1-15 (1999).

[6] Leshnower BG, Kanemoto S, Matsubara M, Sakamoto H, Hinmon R, Gorman JH III, Gorman RC. Cyclosporine Preserves Mitochondrial Morphology After Myocardial Ischemia/ Reperfusion Independent of Calcineurin Inhibition. Ann Thorac Surg, 86; 1286-1292: (2008).

[7] VanDeripe DR. The swelling of Mitochondria by Nitrogen gas; a possible cause of reperfusion damage. Medical Hypotheses 62; 294-296: (2004).

CHAPTER 3:   Stroke and Heart Attack, Reperfusion Injury.

In 2004 the author published in Medical Hypothesis an article entitled- The swelling of mitochondria from nitrogen gas; a possible cause of reperfusion damage [1]. The data base for that article was PhotoEMA (page 6). Shown therein are three giant mitochondria deemed to be swollen with nitrogen gas. The rationale supporting this conclusion follows. The transparent interior of giant mitochondria #s 1, 2, and 3 is gaseous, not liquid because - 1) the internal milieu is electron transparent, i.e. it absorbed none of the incident electron beam [Radiologist have used air in double contrast studies of the colon as a negative contrast agent since it absorbs almost none of the x-ray beam]. 2) The bubbles in #1 are consistent with a gas, i.e. like soap bubbles. Who has seen a bubble of water in water? 3) In mitochondrion #2 we see a bubble in transit into the interior matrix; water would be expected to diffuse, not be transported as bubbles. 4) The transparent internal matrix of these three mitochondria has pushed the cristae to the periphery and has distorted and fragmented their structure. This indicates that the transparent matrix is not miscible with mitochondrial water or particulates. Concluding that the interior of these mitochondria were full of gas, the question became what gas? Taken from an unanesthetized control rat brain, the choices were oxygen, carbon dioxide or nitrogen. Since the brain was harvested and dropped into fixative at one minute and fifteen seconds post decapitation, it seemed clear that the gas was not oxygen, i.e. by that time oxygen should have been used for residual metabolism and certainly would not be there is such excess. Carbon dioxide should have diffused to, and been taken up by deoxyhemoglobin. By process of elimination, the gas had to be nitrogen.

 As early as 1965 Jennings et al [2] published on the changes in myocardial structure following ischemic injury. They reported that after 60 minutes or more of ischemia in dogs the mitochondria of the heart were grossly altered with loss of cristae and abnormally 'clear' matrices; in some cases their limiting membranes were disrupted. Kloner [3] in studying reflow ('74), reported formation of vacuoles and mitochondrial swelling. Lichtig [4], in reperfused pig hearts, described mitochondrial changes consisting of swelling, disruption of cristae and reduction of matrix. In humans, Ferreira [5] reported on the electron microscopic

(EM) histology before and after reperfusion in coronary artery by-pass surgery in patients. They graded mitochondrial EM findings as 1) early swelling, clearing of mitochondrial matrix density and separation of cristae, 2) increased and more evident swelling, 3) massive swelling, with disruption of cristae, and 4) grade 3 findings plus rupture of inner and outer mitochondrial membranes. The observations of the mitochondrial morphology noted in these publications are similar to those in PhotoEMA. A study was undertaken to assess whether total body nitrogen washout [1] from breathing heliox (30% oxygen/70% helium) might limit some of the reperfusion injury in a rat stroke model, [Pan 6]. The infarct volumes were 36% in the controls versus 4% in the heliox washout group of rats. A repeat study, Pan [7], showed an 85% reduction of infarct volumes, when the heliox was initiated immediately after the arterial occlusion, less so with 30-60 minute delays. An attempt to duplicate this effect of heliox on reperfusion injury in rabbit hearts was reported by Hale [8]. The findings were essentially negative. Two variables which might have influenced this study are a) the significant regions of no-reflow, i.e. the target tissue in that animal model, and b) the possibility that the nitrogen washout system was inadequate. Follow up studies should include an in-line nitrogen gas monitor in the expiratory line. The value of heliox during transport of myocardial infarct (MI) patients may be appreciated by the early (1970) article by Piffare et al [9] wherein dogs subjected to double ligation and severing of the left circumflex artery were studied for cardiac parameters including ventricular fibrillation (VF). In 26 dogs breathing air, 14 (54%) demonstrated VF, whereas 55 dogs breathing 20-80% helium only 8 (11%) showed VF. They attributed this protection mainly to opening of collateral circulation. Based on this data and a report by Crampton [10] on the frequency of coronary death during hospital transport, heliox might have clinical value even without complete nitrogen washout activity. It should be noted [11] that heliox washout of nitrogen requires a gas-tight mask, leak-free system.

REFERENCES:

[1] VanDeripe DR. The swelling of mitochondria from nitrogen gas; a possible cause of reperfusion damage. Medical Hypotheses 62; 292-296: (2004).

[2] Jennings RB, Baum, JH, Herndon PB. Fine structural changes in myocardial ischemic injury. Arch Pathol 79; 135-145: (1965).

[3] Kloner RA, Ganote CE, Whalen DA Jr, Jennings RB. Effect of a Transient Period of Ischemia on Myocardial Cells. Am L Pathol. 74; 399-422: (1974).

[4] Lichtig C, Brooks H. Myocardial ultrastructure and function during progressive early ischemia in the intact heart. J of Thoracic and Cardiovascular Surg. 70; 309-315: (1975).

[5] Ferreira R, Lluesuy S, Milei J, Scordo D, Hourquebie H, Molteni L, de Palma C, Boveris A. Assessment of myocardial oxidative stress in patients after myocardial revascularization. Am Heart J, 115; 307-312: (1988).

[6] Pan Y, Zhang H, VanDeripe D, Cruz-Flores S, Panneton WM. Heliox and oxygen reduce infarct volume in a rat model of focal ischemia. Experimental Nurology 205: 587-590 (2007).

[7] Pan Y, Zhang H, Achyara AB, Cruz-Flores S, Panneton WM. The effect of heliox treatment in a rat model of focal transient ischemia. Neurosci Lett. 497; 144-147: (2011).

[8] Hale SL, VanDeripe DR, Kloner RK. Continuous heliox breathing and the extent of anatomic no-reflow and necrosis following ischemia/reperfusion in the rabbit heart. Open Cardiovasc Med. 8; 1-5: (2014).

[9] Piffare R, Raghunath TK, Vanecko RM, Chua FS, Balis JU, Neville WE. Effect of oxygen and helium mixtures on ventricular fibrillation. J. of Thoracic and Cardiovascular Surg. 60; 648-652: (1970).

[10] Crampton B, Aldrich RF, Gascho JA, Miles JR Jr. Stillerman R. Reduction of prehospital, ambulance and community coronary death rates by the community-wide emergency cardiac care system. Am J Med. 58(2); 151-165: (1975).

[11] Standly TD, Smith HL, Brennan LJ, Wilkins IA, Bradley PG, Barrera Groba C, Davy AJ, Menon DK, Wheeler DW. Roomair dilution of heliox given by facemask. Intensive Care Med. 34(8); 1469-1476: (2008).

CHAPTER 4: Reperfusion injury and protection by anesthetic gases.

Literature on the protective effects of volatile and gaseous anesthetics on ischemic/ reperfusion injury have shown positive efficacy for halothane and isoflurane [1], and also xenon [2]. In addition, the non-anesthetic gases helium, argon, and neon [3] and even hydrogen [4] have demonstrated efficacy. In 2001, the author reported on the mechanisms of action of gas and volatile anesthetics and found that halothane, methoxyflurane, enflurane, isoflurane, and ethyl ether formed gas bubbles which invaded and filled mitochondria in the rat brain. Xenon and nitrous oxide also formed bubbles which generally engulfed mitochondria [5]. Based on these findings it would appear that these anesthetic and non-anesthetic gases act as space occupying protective agents, blocking nitrogen access to the mitochondrial matrix. The findings in [5] led to the publication that nitrogen gas was the cause of reperfusion injury following stroke and heart attack [6]. This was followed by two studies by Pan et al [7,8] which demonstrated that total body nitrogen washout (TBNW) by breathing heliox (30% oxygen/70% helium) decreased the necrotic zone in a rat stroke model.

 Paradoxically, these studies [7,8] identified nitrogen as the cause of reperfusion injury and eliminated it from the test animal groups. Conversely, some of the references [1-4] actually used 30% oxygen/70% nitrogen as the positive infarct control to show efficacy for their test gases, i.e. they included the nitrogen poison which causes the problem in the first place. Why is nitrogen the actual cause of reperfusion injury? For one thing, as the major atmospheric gas it is ever-present in the body and it still remains when reperfusion is established. Only then, can it be washed out from the ischemic region based on a reverse concentration clearance. TBNW means no nitrogen in the reperfusing blood. To the extent that the anesthetic gases may be taken up and retained in mitochondria, they may block nitrogen uptake during the infarct period and when reperfusion is attained they are washed out of ischemic tissues and mitochondria as they are exhaled from the blood.

REFERENCES:

[1] Warltier DC, al-Wathiqui MH, Kampine JP, Schmeling WT. Recovery of contractile function of stunned myocaduium in chronically instrumented dogs is enhanced by halothane or isoflurane. Anesthesiology 69(4); 552-565: (1988).

[2] Mio Y, Hee shim Y, Richards E, Bosnial ZJ, Pagel PS, Bienengraeber M. Xenon Preconditioning: The Role of Prosurvival Signaling, Mitochondrial Permeability Transition and Bioenergetics in Rats. Anesth Analg 108(3); 856-866: (2009).

[3] Pagel PS, Krolikowski JG, Shim YH, Venkatapuram S, Kersten JR, Weihrauch D, Warltier DC, Pratt PF Jr. Noble gases without anesthetic properties protect myocardium against infarction by activating prosurvival signaling kinases and inhibiting mitochondrial permeability transition in vivo. Anesth Analg. 105(3); 562-569: (2007).

[4] Hayashida K, Sano M, Ohsawa I, Shinmura K, Tamaki K, Kimura K, Endo J, Katayama A, Kohsaka S, Makino S, Ohta S, Ogawa S, Fukuda K. Inhalation of hydrogen gas reduces infarct size in the rat model of myocardial ischemia-reperfusion injury. Biochem Biophys Res Commun. 373(1); 30-35: (2008).

[5] VanDeripe DR. Gas Microbubbles in Biology: their relevance in Histology, Toxicology, Physiology and Anesthesia. Toxicology Methods 11; 107-126: (2001).

[6] VanDeripe DR. The swelling of mitochondria by Nitrogen gas; a possible cause of reperfusion damage. Med Hypothesis 62; 294-296: (2004)

[7] Pan Y, Zhang H, VanDeripe D, Cruz-Flores, Panneton W. Heliox and oxygen reduce infarct volume in a rat model of focal ischemia. Exp. Neurology 205; 587-590: (2007).

[8] Pan Y, Zhang H, Acharya A, Cruz-Flores S, Panneton W. The effect of heliox treatment in a rat model of focal transient cerebral ischemia. Neurosci Lett. 497; 144-147: (2011).

CHAPTER 5: Other conditions wherein nitrogen gas may exhibit toxicity.

Coronary Artery By-Pass Surgery: It is my understanding from talks with cardiologists that it is not uncommon for CABG patients to exhibit temporary post-surgical mentation problems. It seems reasonable to assume that during the off-pump period patients may experience a degree of mitochondrial compromise in some white matter brain tissue. If this occurs it should be a rather simple experiment to have the patient breath heliox in a tent or one-way mask system to flush out nitrogen from the body during recovery. Alternatively, one might consider switching to heliox prior to surgery on order to eliminate nitrogen effects completely.

Coma or Vegetative State: Could part of these syndromes result from mitochondrial poisoning by nitrogen? Maybe it has already been tried, but if not, total body nitrogen washout may be worth a try.

Serious Injuries: In serious injuries where atrial blood flow leakage in a tissue has to be obtunded for a period of time to allow for surgical repair, a post-surgical total body heliox washout may be in order to eliminate that nitrogen trapped in the ischemic tissue mitochondria.

Gas Gangrene: Chi [1] reported on gases found in a diabetic patient's muscle in gas gangrene. The results were 5.9% hydrogen, 3.4% carbon dioxide, 16.1% oxygen and 74.5% nitrogen. Although oxygen and nitrogen levels approach atmospheric concentrations, that is an extremely high value for nitrogen. Based on water solubility alone nitrogen should be about half that of oxygen. ~8%. This may reflect 'massive' uptake of nitrogen into mitochondria which would lead to the vicious spiral of mitochondrial, cell and tissue death. Total body washout with heliox might mitigate some of the tissue injury if caught early in the infection.

[1] Chi CH, Chen KW, Huang JJ, Chaung YC, Wu MHJ. Gas composition in Clostridium septicum gas gangrene. J. Formos Med Assoc. 94(12); 757-759: (1995).

CHAPTER 6:   Autism Spectrum Disorder (ASD)

What do we know?

- The brain is oversized at two years of age [1, 2] which persists to at least age thirteen [3].
- The cause of this rapid growth is likely due to elevated levels of growth related hormones [4].
- The choroid plexus contains he highest amount of growth hormone receptors in the brain. This suggests a possible transport mechanism for increased supply of growth related hormones by the cerebrospinal fluid (CSF) to target cells in/on the brain surface [5, 6].
- The volume of the ventricles in autistic subjects is higher than controls even when adjusted for intracranial volume [7].
- Increased capillary transit time heterogeneity (slow blood flow) can reduce the oxygen extraction efficiency in brain tissue [8].
- Cerebral blood flow is decreased in autism [9-24].
- There is excess CSF in early autism at 6-24 months which persists to at least 9 years of age [1,36].
- The diameter of the optic nerve sheath is a sensitive indicator of elevated intracranial pressure (ICP) [25-31].

Commentary: What causes autism?

Perhaps it is simply the result of inadequate blood flow to the brain. Increased ICP negatively and in some cases critically inhibits cerebral blood flow. How? The three main contributors to the volume in the skull are 1), the brain per se, 2) the arterial and venous blood volumes, and 3) the volume of CSF. Taken together these three volumes make up the contents which contribute to the ICP. Since we can't reasonably excise some of the brain in order to reduce ICP, we are left with adjustments between blood and CSF volumes to provide optimum brain function and maturation. Simply put, the greater the CSF volume, the less available for blood volume. The critical determinant here is ICP. As ICP rises, blood flow decreases. Nominally the blood pressure drop across the capillary bed is 30 mmHg from arterioles to 10mmHg veins, resulting in a perfusion pressure head of 20 mmHg. Any ICP above 10mmHg is elevated and 20 mmHg is the highest pressure consistent with a 'normal' range in idiopathic normal pressure hydrocephalus [32]. However, in a young autistic child, a 20 mmHg ICP would compress the outer walls of tissue capillaries to an extent that the perfusion pressure only drops from 30 down to 20 mmHg, i.e. a 10 mmHg pressure head equal to 50% of normal. In essence then, the brain blood flow would be cut in half, and is therefore abnormal. It must be appreciated that, unlike peripheral tissues where some stretching is possible, the blood vessels and all tissues of the brain are subjected to identical ICP, and the ICP and CSF pressures become the same. Therefore, too much CSF increases ICP and depresses cerebral blood flow. Non-invasive methodology for evaluating ICP [25-31] utilizes the optic nerve sheath diameter (ONSD) which provides a semi-quantifiable index of ICP. My grandson suffers from ASD and he has ONSD values of 5.84mm and 5.81mm. Geeraerts reports that ONSD values greater than 5.82mm are consistent with ICPs >20mmHG. Elevation of the arterial pressure to 'restore' blood flow in the presence of high ICP may result in thoroughfare shunts and thereby further decrease capillary flow [33]. Ostergaard [8] reports that increased capillary transit time can reduce oxygen extraction into brain tissue. Herbert [34] describe an outer zone of 'radiate' white matter [34] and this may suggest an increased level of tissue CSF and may be more sensitive to poor delivery of oxygen and glucose [35]. This type of water has also been reported by Hendry in T2 MRI studies [36]. (see also Alzheimer's Chapter 7).

Treatment Options:

At this time three options are available for lowering ICP and therein permit increased cerebral blood flow. First is shunting of CSF from the cerebral ventricles to the peritoneal or plural cavities, but this becomes too invasive and problematic for young children. A second option is the use of furosemide, a potent diuretic, which has been used successfully with acetazolamide to lower elevated ICPs greater than 30 mmHg [37]. Although this combination might be considered for initial therapy, a carbonic anhydrase inhibitor such as acetazolamide or some lesser potent agent would be selected for chronic therapy. Extended time 4-14 day dosing with acetazolamide at 50-75 mg/kg infants (~8 Kg) decreased CSF production by 39 and 48% respectively [38]. These time frames suggest that effective levels might be established within one or two months for autism patients presenting with elevated ICP. Diagnosis and monitoring of elevated ICPs might prove to be possible with minimal sedation by employing 1-3 second MRI scans on 3 Tesla magnet equipment.[31]. Note that Lai [5] suggests that CSF may carry certain growth factors (over the brain surface?) to target cells in the brain. That begs the speculative question: Could decreasing the CSF output in very young ASD patients also slow the delivery of growth factors resulting in a slowing of brain growth to a more normal rate? This would assume that growth hormone factors might be secreted at a rate/concentration commensurate with CSF production. If so, early intervention with carbonic anhydrase inhibitors might help to decrease CSF output to a level which slows brain growth.

REFERENCES:

[1] Shen MD, Nordahl CW, Young GS, Wootton-Gorges SL, Lee A, Liston SE, Harrington KR, Ozonoff S, Amaral DG. Early brain enlargement and elevated extra-axial fluid in infants who develop autism spectrum disorder. Brain 136; 2825-2835: (2013).

[2[Hazlett HC, Poe M, Gerig G, Smith RG, Provenzale J, Ross A, Gilmore J, Piven J. Magnetic Resonance Imaging and Head Circumference Study of Brain Size in Autism, Arch Gen Psychiatry 62(1); 1366-1376: (2005).

[3] Piven J, Arndt S, Bailey J, Havercamp S, Andreasen NC, Palmer P. An MRI Study of Brain Size in Autism. Am J. Psychiatry 152; 1145-1149: (1995).

[4] Mills JL, Hediger ML, Molloy CA, Chrousos GP, Manning-Courtney P, Yu KF, Brasington M, England LJ. Elevated levels of growth-related hormones in autism and autism spectrum disorder. Clin Endocrinol (oxf) 67(2); 230-237: (2007).

[5] Lai ZN, Emter M, Roos P, Nyberg F. Characterization of putative growth hormone receptors in human choroid plexus. Brain Res. 546(2); 222-226: (1991).

6] Stopa EG, Berzin TM, Kim S, Song P, Kuo-LeBlanc V, Rodriguez-Wolf M, Baird A, Johanson CE. Human choroid plexus growth factors: What are the implications for CSF dynamics in Alzheimer's disease? Exp Neurol 167(1); 40-47: (2001).

[7] Hardan AY, Minshew NJ, Mallikarjuhn M, Keshavan MS. Brain Volume in autism. J.Child Neurol. 16(6); 421-424: (2001).

[8] Ostergaard L, Jesperson SN, Mouridsen K, Mikkelsen IK, Jonsdottir KY, Tietze A,Blicher JU, Aamand R, Hjort N, Iversen NK, Cai C, Hougaard KD, Simonsen CZ, Von Weitzel-Murdersbach P, Modrau B, Nagenthiraja K, Riisgaard RL, Hansen MB, Bekke SL, Dahlman MG, Puig J, Pedraza S, Serena J, Cho TH, Seimonsen S, Thomalla G, Fiehler H, Nighoghossian N, Andersen G. The role of the cerebral capillaries in acute ischemic srtroke: the extended penumbra model. J. Cereb Blood Flow Metab. (2013).

[9] Gupta SK, Ratnam BV. Cerebral perfusion abnormalities in children with autism and mental retardation: a segmental quantitative SPECT study. Indian Pediatr. 46(2); 161-164: (2009).

[10] Degrirmenci B, Miral S, Kaya GC, Iyillikci L, Arsian G, Baykara A, Evren I, Durak H. Technetium-99m HMPAO brain SPECT in autistic children and their families. Psychriatry Res. 162(3); 236-243: (2008).

[11] Burroni L, Orsi A, Monti L, Hayek Y, Rocchi R, Vattimo AG, Regional cerebral blood flow in childhood autism: a SPET study with SPM evaluation. Nucl Med Commun 29(2); 150-156: (2008).

[12] Ito H, Mori K, Hashimoto T, Miyazaki M, Hori A, Kagami S, Kuroda Y. Findings of brain 99mTc-ECD SPECT in high functioning autism--3- dimensional stereotactic ROI template analysis of brain SPECT. J Med Invest. 52(1-2); 49-56: (2005).

[13] Gendry Meresse I, Zilbovicius M, Boddaert N, Robel L, Philippe A, Sfaello I, Laurier L, Brunelle F, Samson Y, Mouren MC, Chabane N. Autsum severity and temporal lobe functional abnormalities. Ann Neurol. 58(3); 466-469: (2005).

[14] Wilcox J, Tsuang MT, Ledger E, Algeo J, Schnurr T. Brain Perfusion in Autism Varies with Age. Neuropsychobiology 46; 13-16: (2002).

[15] Boddaert N Zilbovicius M. Functional neuroimaging and childhood autism. Pediatr Radiol. 32(1); 1-7: (2002).

[16] Galuska L, Szakall S Jr, Emri M, Olah R, Varga J, Garai I, Kollar J, Pataki I, Tron L. PET and SPECT scans in autistic children. Orv. Hetil 143(21 Suppl 3); 1302-1304: (2002).

[17] Kaya M, Karasalihoglu S, Ustun F, Gultekin A, Cermik TF, Fazlioglu Y, Ture M, Yigitbasi ON, Berkarda S. The relationship between 99mTc-HMPAO brain SPECT and the scores of real life rating scale in autistic children. Brain Dev. 24(2); 77-81: (2002}.

[18] Boddaert N, Chabane N, Barthelemy C,, Bourgeois M, Poline JB, Brunelle F, Samson Y, Zilbovicius M. Bitemporal lobe dysfonction in infantile autism: positron emission tomography study. J. Radiol. 83 (12 Pt 1); 1829-1833: (2002).

[19] Hashimoto T, Sasaki M, Fukumizu M, Hanaoka S, Sugai K, Matsuda H, Single-photon emission tomography of the brain in autism: effect of the developmental level. Pediater Neurol. 23(5); 416-420: (2000).

[20] Ziilbovicius M, Boddaert N, Belin P, Poline JB, Remy P, Mangin JF, Thivard L, Barthelemy C, Samson Y. Temporal lobe dysfunction in childhood autism: a PET study. Positron emission tomography. Am J Psychiatry 157(12); 1988-1993: (2000).

[21] Onishi T, Matsuda H, Hashimoto T, Kunihiro T, Nishikawa M, Uema T, Sasaki M. Abnormal regional cerebral blood flow in childhood autism. Brain 123(pt9); 1838-1844: (2000).

[22] Ryu YH, Lee JD, Yoon PH, Kim DI, Lee HB, Shin YJ. Perfusion impairments in infantile autism on technetium-99m ethyl cysteinate dimer brain single-photon emission tomography: comparison with findings on magnetic resonance imaging. Eur J Nucl Med. 26(3); 253-259: (1999).

[23] Mountz JM, Tolbert LC, Lill DW, Katholi CR, Liu HG. Functional deficits in autistic disorder: characterization by technetium-99m-HMPAO and SPECT. J Nucl Med. 36(7); 1156-1162: (1995).

[24] Carina Gillberg I, Bjure J, Uvebrant P, Vestergren E, Gillberg C. SPECT (Single Photon Emission Computed Tomography) in 31 children and adolescents with autism and autistic-like conditions. Eur Child Adolesc Psychiatry. 2(1); 59-59: (1993).

[25] Watanabe A, Kinouchi H, Horikoshi T, Uchida M, Ishigame K. Effect of intracranial pressure on the diameter of the optic nerve sheath. J Neurosurg 109; 255-258: (2008).

[26] Geeraerts T, Newcombe VFJ, Coles JP, Abate MG, Perkes LE, Hutchinson PJA, Outtrim JG, Chatfield DA, Manon DK. Use of T2-weighted magnetic resonance imaging of the optic nerve sheath to detect raised intracranial pressure. Crit Care 12(5); R114: (2008).

[27] Kimberly HH, Noble VE, Using MRI of the optic nerve sheath to detect elevated intracranial pressure. Crit Care 12(5); 181 (2008).

[28] Geeraerts T, Dubost C, Theme: Neurology-Optic nerve sheath diameter measurement as a risk marker for significant intracranial hypertension. Biomarkers in Medicine 3.2; 129: (2009).

[29] Xie X, Zhang X, Fu J, Wang H, Jonas JB, Peng X, Tian G, Xian J, Ritch R, Li L, Kang Z, Zhang S, Tang D, Wang N. Noninvasive intracranial pressure estimation by orbital subarachnoid space measurement: the Beijing Intracranial and Intraocular Pressure (iCOP) study. Crit Care 17(4) R162 (2013).

[30] Geeraerts T, Noninvasive surrogates of intracranial pressure: another piece added with magnetic resonance imaging of the cerebrospinal fluid thickness surrounding the optic nerve. Crit Care 17(5); 187 (2013).

[31] Weigel M, Lagreze WA, Lazzaro A, Hennig J, Blay TA. Fast and Quantitative High-Resolution Magnetic Resonance Imaging of the Optic Nerve at 3.0 Tesla. Invest Radiol. 41; 83-86: (2006).

[32] Savolainen S, Paljarvi L, Vapalahti, Prevalence of Alzheimer's Disease in Patients Investigated for Presumed Normal Pressure Hydrocephalus: A Clinical and Neuropathological Study. Arch Neurochir (Wien) 141; 849-853 (1999).

[33] Bragin DE, Bush RC, Muller WS, Nemoto EM. High intracranial pressure effects on cerebral cortical microvascular flow in rats. J Neurotrauma 28(5) 775-785 (2011).

[34] Herbert MR, Ziegler DA, Makris N, Filipek PA, Kemper TL, Normandin JJ, Kennedy DN, Caviness VS Jr. Localization of white matter volume increase in autism and developmental language disorder. Ann Neurol 55(4); 530-540: (2004).

[35] Kalback W, Esh C, Castano EM, Rahman A, Kokjohn T, Lurhrs DC, Sue L, Cisneros R, Gerber F, Richardson C, Bohrmann B, Walker DG, Beach TG, Roher AE. Atherosclerosis, vascular hypoperfusion in the pathogenesis of sporadic Alzheimer's disease. Neurol Res. 26; 525-539: (2004).

[36] Hendry J. DeVito T Gelman N, Densmore M, Rajakumar N, Pavlosky W, Williamson PC, Thompson PM, Drost DJ, Nicolson R. White matter abnormalities in autism detected through transverse relaxation time imaging. Neuroimage. 29(4); 1049-1057: (2006).

[37] Schoeman JF. Childhood Pseudotumor Cerebri: Clinical and Intracranial Pressure Response to Acetazolamide and Furosemide Treatment in a case series. J. Child Neurol 9: 130-134: (1994).

[38] Carrion E, Hertzog JH, Medlock MD, Hauser GJ, Dalton HJ, Use of acetazolamide to decrease cerebrospinal fluid production in chronically ventilated patients with ventriclopleural shunts. Arch Dis Child. 84(1); 68-71: (2001).

CHAPTER 7:   Alzheimer's disease (AD)

Perhaps AD is mainly a disease of deficient cerebral blood flow which may result from a number of factors which eventually combine and progress to the clinical 'disease'. Causes of reduced blood flow to the brain are summarized by de la Torre [1] and include advancing age and vascular risk factors. Kalback [2] specifies vascular risk factors to be atherosclerosis and vascular amyloidosis which cause a decrease in perfusion pressure. Wegiel [3] points to vascular fibrosis and calcification in the hippocampus during aging. Farkas indicates that it is well known that the brain is particularly vulnerable to suboptimal oxygen and glucose delivery (4). Specific blood flow issues have been attributed to the CA-1 region of the hippocampus [West 5], [deLeon 6] where the earliest histological neuronal loss has been reported. Marinkovic [7] reports that the most sensitive part of the hippocampal formation is the CA-1 sector also known as the Sommer's sector. The basis of this sensitivity difference may lie in the fact that the CA-1 sector is supplies by one large (ventral) artery. Other areas are supplied not only by one large (dorsal) artery, but also by other smaller vessels. As well, the CA-1 sector has a smaller number of microvessels than the other hippocampal sectors. The specific characteristics of the metabolism and the membrane receptors of the CA-1 pyramidal neurons may be a main reason for their higher sensitivity to ischemia. Marinkovic lists the diameters of middle hippocampal artery as ranging from 310-800 microns with a mean value of 588 microns. To the extent that insufficiency could develop over time, the smaller (310 micron) vessels would have less flow redundancy and become candidates for causing mitochondrial hypoxia, leading to mitochondrial 'apoptosis', cell and tissue death. This would result in cellular debris which could plug the arachnoid villi and result in increased cerebrospinal fluid (CSF) and intracranial pressure (ICP). Vascular fibrosis and calcification in the middle hippocampus artery and capillary network results in patchy neuronal loss in moderately affected subjects [Weigel 3]. West [6] reports that the CA-1 segment of the hippocampus from an AD group contained 4.4 million neurons versus 14.1 million in a normal control group.

Kalback [2] studied white matter from AD vs age matched controls and found that white matter from AD cases was soft, friable and easily deformed under pressure. In contrast, white matter from elderly controls was firmer, denser and of resilient consistency. In addition, the white matter atrophy and enlarged ventricles are both impressive features of AD. As well, another major difference in AD is the more frequent and noticeable enlargement of white matter perivascular spaces. They stated that their interest in studying pathological alterations in AD originated from the observation that approximately two-thirds of the cases demonstrated areas of white matter rarefaction. These regions have significant loss of myelin, oligodendroglia and a considerable deficit of microvessels resulting in a severe hypoxia of the white matter. The normal white matter is largely substituted by swollen astrocytes and edema. From a hemodynamic point of view, both amyloidosis and atherosclerosis reduce cerebral blood flow and increase the pulse index indicative of reduced arterial compliance and peripheral resistance. As expected the most severe microvascular and blood brain barrier damage would be localized in the most distal regions of the brain's arterial network, i.e. deep white matter. In electron microscopic photos, Kalback compares AD to normal and notes that in AD, white matter oligodendrocytes, myelin, and axons have been replaced with interstitial water and swollen and large astrocytes. Perhaps these findings bring into focus the MRI –T2 white matter hyperintensities (WMH) reported by Carmichael et al [8], in which the WMH volume was associated with one year cognitive decline in AD. Kalback's histology suggests that the WMH may actually represent dying or mostly dead tissue loaded with interstitial water which accounts for the enhanced T2 signals. This water may be CSF which has invaded dead tissue.

A nonvascular participant in the skull of the AD subject which has received scant attention in the literature is cerebrospinal fluid (CSF) volume and which interacts and contributes to intracranial pressure (ICP) to an extent that they become essentially equivalent. Condon [9] reported that MRI imaging found the lateral ventricle and intracranial CSF volumes to be 25ml and 98ml respectively in normal and 53ml and 151ml in a patent with cerebral atrophy due to AD. Three factors might account for the increased CSF volume: 1) simple replacement of volume left from dead brain tissue, 2) excess production of CSF by the choroid plexuses, or 3) Silverberg [10] decreased resorption of CSF by the arachnoid villi system, possibly due to increased outflow resistance caused by fibrosis of the arachnoid tissue. Savolainen [11] investigated patients with presumed normal pressure hydrocephalus (NPH) and noted histological evidence from cerebral biopsies indicating that 50-118 (42%) were consistent with AD based on the presence of plaques, amyloid load and tau protein. These findings along with higher levels of CSF, decrease blood flow to the point that increased ICP may play a role as a causative factor in the development of AD. Now that ICP can be detected and somewhat quantified by MRI measurement of the optic nerve sheath diameter (ONSD) [see articles by Geeraerts and others in Autism chapter] consideration of early and routine monitoring of ONSD should be implemented in the at-risk AD population. Elevated ICP might well be treatable by administration of carbonic anhydrase inhibitor therapeutic agents such as acetazolamide. Lowering the ICP may permit an improved blood flow to white matter and thereby lessen and/or delay the development of AD. Note that an ICP of 20 mmHg might reduce capillary blood flow by about 50% and double the capillary blood transit time, which may adversely affect the transport of oxygen and glucose across capillary membranes [12]. Also, increased capillary transit time heterogeneity can trigger a critical lack of oxygen in brain tissue [13]. Decreased cerebral perfusion pressure with increased ICP is likely due to redistribution of microvascular shunt flow or thoroughfare shunt channels [14]. Appearance of fibroblast growth factor receptors in AD arachnoid was associated with robust amyloid and vimentin immunoreactivity which suggests that the arachnoid villi complex may be partially plugged and require higher ICP to filter and resorb CSF into the venous drainage [15].

Finally, de la Torre [1], states that last and most important, recent studies suggest that regional hypometabolism measured in AD brains does not appear to result from neurodegenerative changes but appears to precede it. This is probably the most important 'axiom' regarding AD. Many of the above observations are the results of the condition, not its cause. It becomes irreversible, so one must treat it early as soon as significant symptoms are detectable. To this end detecting raised ICP and lowering it to reach levels of 10 mmHg or even perhaps somewhat lower may delay many of the circulatory, mitochondrial and tissue death issues. In support for the therapy to reduce ICP in AD, an article by Akiguchi et al [16] warrants attention. The topic is shunt-responsive parkinsonism. In a study of 17 definitive idiopathic normal pressure hydrocephalus patients, 15 (88%) demonstrated white matter lesions on their CT or MRI images. These signs were ameliorated after shunting. Clinically the patients had frequent parkinsonism (71%). Over half also showed signs of cognitive impairment and urinary incontinence and all such symptoms improved significantly after shunting. What does shunting of CSF accomplish? It decreases the volume of CSF in the skull. Could that alone reverse the signs of parkinsonism. Yes because removing CSF lowers ICP which could enhance capillary blood flow to 'ischemic' tissue. The same might be expected for AD.

In Chapter 19, I propose an omnibus ~$ three million study on Alzheimer's with special attention to measurements of the optic nerve sheath diameters for estimations of intracranial pressure (ICP). It occurs to me reading the article of Carmichael [8], that the ICP data may already be 'out there' in the original T2 MRI images. They stripped non brain tissue from their image analysis. Therefore, T2 images of the eyes, optic nerves and optic nerve sheaths were likely omitted. If so, they could retrieve the original T2 images and measure the optic nerve sheath diameters as reported by Geeraerts and others [see references 25-31 in chapter 6]. Then, if significant elevation of ICP is supported by ONSD measurements in the 804 patient study group, the omnibus study is justified. However, if no ICP elevations are found, the concept of acetazolamide therapy to reduce ICP in Alzheimer's is moot.

REFERENCES:

[1] de la Torre JC. Impaired Cerebrovascular Perfusion: Summary of Evidence in Support of its Causality in Alzheimer's Disease. Annals New York Academy of Sciences 924; 136-152: (2000).

[2] Kalback W, Esh C, Castano EM, Rahman A, Kokjohn T, Luehrs DC, Sue L, Cisneros R, Gerber F, Richardson C, Bohrmann B, Walker DC, Beach TG, Roher AE. Atherosclerosis, vascular amyloidosis and brain hypoperfusion in the pathogenesis of sporadic Alzheimer's disease. Neurol Res. 26; 525-539: (2004).

[3] Wegiel J, Kuchna I, Wisniewski T, de Leon MJ, Reisberg B, Pittila T, Kivmaki T, Lehtimaki T. Vascular fibrosis and calcification in the hippocampus in aging, Alzheimer disease, and Down syndrome. Acta Neuropathol 103(4); 333-343: (2002).

[4] Farkas E, DeJong GI, Apro E, DeVos RA, Steur EN, Luiten PG. Similar ultrastructure breakdown of cerebrocortical capillaries in Alzheimer's disease, Parkinson's disease, and experimental hypertension. What is the functional link? Ann N Y Acad Sci. 903; 72-82: (2000).

[5] West MJ, Coleman PD, Flood DG, Troncoso JC. Differences in the pattern of hippocampal loss in normal ageing and Alzheimer's disease. Lancet 344(8925); 769-772: (1994).

[6] de Leon MJ, Convit A, DeSanti S, Bobinski M, George AE, Wisniewski HM, Rusinek H, Carroll R, Saint Louis LA. Contribution of structural neuroimaging to the early diagnosis of Alzheimer's disease. Int Psychogeriatr. 9 Suppl 1; 183-190 (discussion) 247-252: (1997).

[7] Marinkovic S, Milisavljevic M, Puskas L. Microvascular Anatomy of the Hippocampal Formation. Surg Neurol 37; 339-349: (1992).

[8] Carmichael O, Schwarz C, Drucker D, Fletcher E, Harvey D, Beckett L, Jack CR, Weiner M, DeCarli C. Longitudinal Changes in White Matter Disease and Cognition in the First Year of the Alzheimer Disease Neuroimaging Initiative. Arch Neurol 67(11); 1370-1378: (2010).

[9] Condon B, Patterson J, Wyper D, Hadley D, Grant R, Teasdale G, Rowan J. Use of magnetic resonance imaging to measure intracranial cerebrospinal fluid volume. Lancet 1 (8494); 1355-1357: (1986).

[10] Silverberg G, Mayo M, Saul T, Fellmann J, McGuire D. Elevated cerebrospinal fluid pressure in patients with Alzheimer's disease. Cerebrospinal Fluid Res. 3; 7: (2006).

[11] Savolainen S, Paljarvi I, Vapalahti M. Prevalence of Alzheimer's Disease in Patients Investigated for Presumed Normal Pressure Hydrocephalus: A Clinical and Neuropathological Study. Arch Neurchir (Wien) 141; 849-853: (1999).

[12] Tang Z, Pi X, Chen F, Shi L, Gong H, Fu H, Qu Z. Fifty Percent Reduced-Dose Cerebral CT Perfusion Imaging of Alzheimer's Disease: Regional Blood Flow Abnormalities. Am J Alzheimers Dis Other Demen. 27(4); 267-274: (2012).

[13] Ostergaard L, Jespersen SN, Mouridsen K, Mikkelsen IK, Jonsdottir KY, Tietze A, Blicher JU, Aamand R, Hjort N, Iversen NK, Cai C, Hougaard KD, Simonsen CZ, Von Weitzel-Mudersbach P, Modrau B, Nagenthiraja K, Riisgaard RL, Hansen MB, Bekke SL, Dahlman MG, Puig J, Pedraza S, Serena J, Cho TH, Siemonsen S, Thomalla G, Fiehler J, Nighoghossian N, Andersen G. The role of the cerebral capillaries in acute ischemic stroke: the extended penumbra model. J. Cereb Blood Flow Metab. 33(5); 635-648: (2013).

[14] Bragin DE, Bush RC, Mullar WS, Nemoto EM. High intracranial pressure effects on cerebral cortical microvascular flow in rats. J. Neurotrauma 28(5); 775-785: (2011).

[15] Stopa EG, Berzin TM, Kim S, Song P, Kuo-LeBlanc V, Rodriguez-Wolf M, Baird A, Johanson CE. Human choroid plexus growth factors: What are the implications for CSF dynamics in Alzheimer's disease? Exp Neurol 167(1); 40-47: (2001).

[16] Akiguchi I, Ishii M, Watanabe Y, Watanabe T, Kawasaki T, Yagi H, Shiino A, Shirakashi Y, Kawamoto Y. Shunt-responsive parkinsonism and reversible white matter lesions in patients with idiopathic NPH. J. Neurol 255; 1392-1399: (2008).

Chapter 8: CNS disease, the bowling ball hypothesis

de la Torre [1] reported in Chapter 7, "last and most important, recent studies suggest that regional hypometabolism in Alzheimer's disease brains does not appear to result from neurodegenerative changes but appears to precede it."

This clearly points to an inadequate effort to identify and correct to the extent possible the causes of hypometabolism, which must be preceded by an understanding of the causes and role of regional hypoperfusion of the brain. In short, there may be regions in the brain that simply do not get enough oxygen.

Unlike the rest of the body, the blood flow to the brain is limited because of the skull. Let us imagine the skull as a hollowed out bowling ball with a wall of about one centimeter thickness and the three holes would represent 1) the thumb hole would be the outgoing (efferent) spinal cord, meninges, spinal fluid, etc. 2) a finger hole as another efferent drains the venous blood, cerebrospinal fluid (CSF) from the arachnoid villi complex, and lymph, etc., and 3) the second finger hole is the incoming (afferent) arterial blood vessels and blood supply, which gives rise to the choroid plexuses which becomes a second afferent as it secretes CSF into the cranial cavity. Therefore, it becomes clear that the three players in the skull are the volumes of brain, blood and CSF. Accepting that the brain is allowed to keep its space (volume), we then are limited to downward adjustments in CSF volume if we can hope to increase brain blood flow. Decreasing CSF volume has been conducted mainly by shunting of CSF from the lateral ventricles into the peritoneal or pleural cavities. This has worked to some degree, but infection and plugged systems have often been problematic. Reducing the production of CSF by the use of carbonic anhydrase inhibitor drugs has been proven effective, but again with mixed results.

 So, what are some of the details and which ones may be amenable to some level of control. First, let us consider the vascular component. Blood vessel growth and development to the brain is generally consistent up to and perhaps for one or two declinations beyond the Circle of Willis. Beyond this however, we get into abnormal deviation regions of the bell shape normal distribution curve. Two studies which tend to support this concept are Marinkovic [2] and Uz [3].

Marinkovic, measured the diameter of the middle hippocampal artery in 25 specimensand reported values ranging from 310-800 microns with a mean value of 588 microns. Uz measured the diameter of the anterior choroidal artery in 15 fresh cadavers and reported values from 0.7mm to 1.2mm with a mean value of 0.94mm. To the degree that these samples may represent the total population, one might surmise that the 310 micron and 0.7mm diameters might represent vessels with very little built-in redundancy with respect to downstream blood flow. Therefore, with aging, they would be candidates for progressively declining blood flows due to factors such as smoking and atherosclerosis to further decrease vessel lumens, and as well, the physiological declines in cardiac output and increasing pulse pressure which, in smaller vessels, might begin to approach a water hammer pulse with greatly diminished diastolic blood flow. Over time, this will result in an inadequate delivery of oxygen to mitochondria and a diminished production of adenosine triphosphate, leading to a slow, but relentless, 'increasing percentage' pumping of nitrogen into mitochondria by the mitochondrial permeability transitions pore (mPTP). Finally mitochondrial function will cease via apoptotic or necrotic pathways, leading to cell and tissue death. Then will follow all of the 'scar' tissues such as plaques, tangles, tau protein, etc.

If we are to successfully treat Alzheimer's, and other related diseases e.g. Parkinson's, Huntingtons Chorea, ALS, and generalized dementia, we must start early, because limited reversibility is possible, i.e. dead brain tissue is dead forever. Two approaches, which should probably be combined, are to increase blood flow and breathing nitrogen-free air. If general brain blood flow is the problem its significance may be detected by measurement of Intracranial pressure (ICP). See chapter 6 (Autism) for a series of articles reporting on the value of MRI imaging of the optic nerve sheath diameter as a means of semi-quantifying ICP. If ICPs of CNS disease candidates are elevated above about 10mmHg, then acetazolamide or other carbonic anhydrase inhibitors should be considered as an approach lower CSF production and thereby elevate cerebral blood flow. Since the normal drop in pressure across the capillary bed is about 30mmHg (arteriolar) down to 10mmHg (collecting veins) resulting in a perfusion pressure of 20mmHg, any ICP above 10mmHg will adversely impact blood flow and it will become progressively worse as ICP approaches 20mmHg. Certainly, in normal physiology the brain has a capability to redistribute blood as needed to various regions of the brain. But, in the case of elevated ICPs, physics trumps physiology. The second approach, breathing nitrogen free air is valid based on the mitochondrial toxicity of nitrogen during ischemia/anoxia. The extent to which the breathing of nitrogen-free air is applicable depends on the condition being treated. As detailed in chapters 2-5 there are some acute conditions with temporary blood flow cessation, e.g. stroke, heart attack etc., wherein the breathing of heliox (nominally 30%oxygen/70% helium) may only require 2-3 hours to provide total body nitrogen washout (TBNW) in order to protect mitochondrial function. However, in the chronic CNS diseases the required breathing periods may be continual, i.e. a 24 hour artificial nitrogen free environment. More likely, however, would be that daily or even weekly schedules for one-two hours of TBNW would be developed to prevent/minimize mitochondrial apoptosis/death.

References:

[1] de la Torre JC. Impaired Cerebrovascular Perfusion: Summary of Evidence in Support of its Causality in Alzheimer's Disease. Annals New York Academy of Sciences 924; 136-152: (2000).

[2] Marinkovic SW, Milisavljevic M, Puskas L. Microvascular Anatomy of the Hippocampal Formation. Surg Neurol 37; 339-349: (1992).

[3] Uz A, Erbil KM, Esmer AF. The origin and relations of the anterior choroidal artery: an anatomical study. Folia Morphol (Warsz) 64; 269-272 (2005).

Chapter 9: Integration of chapters 2 through 7 and nitrogen gas as a poison

First and Foremost----   Nitrogen Gas is an ever-present, opportunistic poison!!

Clearly we are talking about acute, sub-acute and chronic ischemia, and the treatment strategies must allow for these differences. Where the insult is acute such as in heart attack or stroke, the potential for reperfusion injury therapies include total body nitrogen washout (TBNW) using heliox initiated early in the ambulance. In the case of stroke, heliox washout of nitrogen most likely would be delayed until CAT scanning would differentiate ischemic vs hemorrhagic stroke; heliox TBNW may not be indicated for the latter.

With respect to Autism Spectrum Disorder and Alzheimer's disease, elevated intracranial pressure (ICP) would trigger the use of carbonic anhydrase inhibitors such as acetazolamide in order to decrease the production of cerebrospinal fluid as a means to reduce ICP and thereby allow an increase in cerebral blood flow. Increased cerebral blood flow in acute and chronic conditions as above will provide more oxygen to mitochondria, thereby blocking nitrogen-mediated mitochondrial apoptosis, cell and tissue death.

As an ongoing maintenance therapy for the above acute and chronic conditions, one might envision the development of 'heliox houses' where rooms would be equipped to provide for atmospheres of ~30% oxygen/70% helium and with nitrogen and carbon dioxide scrubbed during each recirculation. The purpose of such therapy would be a periodic wash out of nitrogen from the body prior to its reaching 'mitochondrial apoptosis' triggering levels. Such prophylactic treatments should minimize mitochondrial swelling/death. Optimum intervals of these therapies would be determined by clinical trial investigations. These heliox house facilities might be open 24 hours per day to provide walk-in TBNW therapy.

Chapter 10: Nitrogen Gas as a chemotherapeutic agent.

IF, the above adverse toxic potential for nitrogen gas can be shown to be a valid biological issue, then we should consider the possibility of its reverse 'therapeutic' value. Simply put, we identify a tumor where the blood supply can be obtunded. Within 2-3 minutes oxygen levels will approach zero and then nitrogen saturated saline will be 'instilled' into the tumor tissue. That nitrogen will be taken up by oxygen starved mitochondria leading to mitochondrial swelling, and on reflow, mitochondria apoptosis and death, tumor cell and tissue death. Too easy??

Chapter 11: Organic Solvents as in vivo therapy for HIV and E Bola.

Now, we get a bit weird...

Has anyone thought about delipidating viruses *in vivo*. Two organic solvents which might be considered would be pentane and ethyl ether. The latter has been reported to have in vitro activity against viruses [1]. To be effective, pentane and ether would have to be present in the liquid state in vivo. Therefore they would need to be gently heated for inhalation and then accumulated in tissues as liquids, which would necessitate cooling of body temperatures to levels slightly lower than the boiling points of these solvents. The boiling point for pentane is 36.2 degrees C, and that for ether is 34.6 degrees C. These temperatures convert to about 97.16F and 94.23F respectively. To have these agents convert back into the liquid state in vivo would only require relatively mild hypothermia in each case. The duration of exposure and dose of these agents for efficacy would be determined by animal experimentation. A note on the safety of ethyl ether. Except for its flammable/explosive potential, ether remains one of the safest anesthetics. Its toxic/lethal dose is at least twice the anesthetic dose. Here, let me comment on a demonstration that Dr. Moran and I performed before a class of Emory medical students on ether's safety. After anesthesia with a short acting barbiturate to prepare a dog for measurement of blood pressure, pulse pressure, heart rate, electrocardiogram, and respiratory rate/depth, we switched over to the administration of ether. We continued the administration of ether until complete respiratory arrest was achieved. All of the above parameters were displayed on a TV screen. We then told the students, yell when you think we need to start artificial respiration. Well, after about 90 seconds when all the functions were still 'perfect' except respiratory arrest, students began to become uneasy and voice concerns – "do something". After another 15-20 seconds, I looked at Dr. Moran, he nodded, and I compressed the chest only twice. The dog began to breath and return toward normal. The point here is that ether is safe when used with care re its flammability.

[1] Quinnan GV Jr, Wells MA, Wittek AE, Phelan MA, Mayner RE, Feinstone S, Purcell RH, Epstein JS. Inactivation of hyman T-cell lymphotropic virus, Type III by heat, chemicals and irradiation. Transfusion 26(5); 481-483 (1986).

Chapter 12: Capsule comments from 2001 publication on anesthesia

It is probable that few anesthesiologists have read my paper; Gas Microbubles in Biology: Their Relevance in Histology, Toxicology, Physiology and Anesthesia. Toxicology Methods 11(2); 107-126: (2001). The main reason may be that PubMed never picked it up in their title/abstract service. I tried to get them to include Toxicology Methods in their 'library', but was told it wasn't on the list. So now, as of March of 2015 it has been available. Go to Google, Taylor&Francis and the above title.

The question asked was, -could gas and volatile anesthetics act in the form of gas bubbles in vivo? The upshot was yes, and the study also answered several enigmas which existed in 2001. First: Contrary to the Meyer-Overton laws wherein the more lipid soluble the anesthetics in each series have the higher potency, this breaks down in the alkane series. There, pentane is a weak anesthetic, but the more lipid soluble compounds octane and decane have no anesthetic activity. Simply put pentane boils at 36.2 degrees C and will be present as a gas phase at body temperature (37.4C). On the other hand the boiling points of octane (125.6C) and decane (174C) are very high and they would not be present as gases even to trivial extents at body temperature. Second: enflurane and isoflurane are isomers, yet the latter is about half-again more potent than the former. Why? Again, boiling points; enflurane 56.5 and isoflurane 48.5, so at body temperature, more of the isoflurane would exist in the vaporphase than enflurane. Third: Why does Indoklon (fluothyl) evoke convulsions. Fluothyl is hexafluroether. As such it is highly hydrophobic and forms angstrom range sized gas bubbles, similar in size to synaptic vesicles. Therein, both their size and hydrophobicity favor targeting/ disruption of vesicles and release of neurotransmitter. Fourth: Why do gas and volatile anesthetics exhibit an excitement phase which requires premedication? Gas and especially volatile anesthetics form bubbles which surround synaptic vesicles at perhaps >25 vesicles per bubble. This means that the surrounding gas phase will have two effects. First; it will immediately block neurotransmitter re-uptake leading to the excitement phase, and Second; rapid anesthesia develops as transmitter levels drop and further transmitter release is blocked because the nerve signals cannot traverse the gas bubble barrier.

Chapter 13: Exactly, what is a vacuole?

Medical dictionary (Gould) 1049, Vacuole (vacuum); - a clear space in a cell. Well now, that just doesn't cut it (vacuum?). It wouldn't even cut it if it said (vacant). The fact that it is a clear space in a cell indicates that we see it under microscopic conditions. So, since nature abhors a vacuum, it has to be something. And, if it totally transparent, it is almost certainly gaseous. It is not acceptable to infer that it was washed out during the fixation process. My first experience with a vacuole was in Botany Lab looking at a leaf under a microscope. I asked the instructor- what's this? He answered, it is a vacuole, label it so. Years later I thought, what is the function of a leaf? Is it not to carry out photosynthesis, i.e. take up carbon dioxide and give off oxygen? If one assumes that the carbon dioxide is taken up on a molecular level, said vacuole must be an oxygen bubble on its way back to the atmosphere. In Chapter 4, Kloner reports tissue vacuoles in a reperfusion study. One might wonder whether these might not actually represent bubbles of oxygen, delivered to the tissue, but not taken up into mitochondria which are swollen with nitrogen gas?

Chapter 14: Fixatives in Histology.

In the fixation of tissues for electron microscopy, there have been numerous articles published. My only suggestion here is in reference to chapter 3 wherein the tissue fixative used was 2% glutaraldehyde (slightly hypotonic). The advantage of this fixative was that it permitted tissues to retain all of their water and, as a result, also the gas bubbles. A contract laboratory fixative used for comparison (2 fixatives and buffers) was 7.4 hypertonic and flushed nearly all gas bubbles from the specimen via osmotic dehydration. I mention this because it is my impression that many/most labs use somewhat highly buffered fixatives in order to attain the maximum anatomic resolution and detail. This sacrifices any information one might obtain on the presence of tissue gases. Perhaps, fixation of a small portion of biopsies in 2-3% glutaraldehyde might provide useful complementary information.

Chapter 15: All of the above is wrong; gases are soluble in water.

This is an argument that someone is bound to proffer against the tone of this tome. Gases are not soluble in water they are dispersible in water. If they were soluble in water, they should travel down diffusion gradients such that oxygen would find its way into ischemic tissues and mitigate almost all of the tissue damaged following strokes and heart attacks. The fact that one can view bubbles in the electron photomicographs of different gas and volatile anesthetic agents and untreated controls rats verifies the presence of gas bubbles (chapter 3). An interesting experiment might be to assemble equipment to include a cold/ freeze stage electron microscope, a one liter beaker, a pipette, an oxygen electrode, a micron sized frit, a small tank of oxygen, and a liter of freshly distilled, gas free water. At room temperature ~25 degrees C, pipette a drop of the water on to the EM viewing stage. No gas, expect sample to appear smooth and the oxygen electrode to read zero. Then start infusing micronized oxygen at one ml per minute into beaker. At about 3% water solubility the oxygen should take about 30 minutes to saturate the 1000ml of water, and minute by minute pipette samples should continue to look smooth on the EM, and the oxygen electrode should record increasing levels of oxygen. Only after this thirty minute period should bubbles be apparent in the beaker and start to show up as 'structural bubble noise' on the EM. If the EM shows said bubble noise within 1 or 2 minutes and the oxygen electrode also shows rising levels, then the oxygen is dispersible, but not soluble.

Chapter 16: Pinocytosis.

My first exposure to pinocytosis, aka cell drinking, was at the 1958 fall meetings of the Phramacology society held at the U. of Michigan. At one of the sessions there was a movie on pinocytosis presented by Chauncey Leake. The movie was a real time microscopic viewing of rat mesentery and the delivery and uptake of bubbles of water in the in the capillary circulation. Uptake was by cells of the capillary endothelium and consisted of an endocytotic 'gobbling-up' of the water. For years, off and on, I have thought about this movie and it goes like this. We see blood in the capillaries and flow is evident. Suddenly there pops up in the capillary lumen a rather large bubble of water which gets gobbled-up. Cell drinking was the call, I say no. First. How does the brain know where to drop off the bubble of water, what is the signaling system, what is the feedback loop, how does the cell tell the brain - I'm thirsty? How the heck does the blood just pop out a bubble of clear transparent water? Why would the bubble of water be crystal clear, we don't have tear glands or ducts in our blood? Why did it not immediately re-mix with plasma? How could a bubble of water remain pure for even one or two seconds? If water, then should not the bubble simply diffuse across the capillary endothelium, why would it be broken-up/gobbled up? The answer is simple physiology. One of the major jobs of the blood is to deliver oxygen to the tissue. Most of this oxygen is bound to hemoglobin. At the level of the capillary, perhaps 10,000 molecules of oxyhemoglobin dump their oxygen at nearly the same time. Individual molecules of oxygen coalesce into one 'large' bubble, which IS transparent, IS not miscible with water, IS not diffusible through the capillary membranes and therefore must be endocytosed. Conclusion: The film was striking demonstration of normal physiology.

OK, why this. Another piece of support that gases are dispersible, but not soluble in the body.

Chapter 17: Where and what is the FOG?

To a degree it is everywhere. Certainly, nothing herein holds a candle to the exotic cures we can expect from genetics, biotechnology, complex biochemistry, bla, bla over the next ten to fifty years. NOTE: The word cure is not used anywhere in this discourse. The entire conceptual framework is better short term therapy. Make the patients suffering from heart attack, stroke, autism, Alzheimer's and other CNS conditions do better.

The FOG is predominantly NIH. NIH means National Institutes of Health, whose expertise coupled with academic advisors put out Requests for Proposals directed at their most important priorities. Well, if they are as far off target as the Congress' spending proposals, God help us! NIH also means, especially in universities- NOT Invented Here. The impetus there is primarily for big dollar federal (other) grants, so they simply don't have time for some short term yes/no programs. There is also some ego controlling the university attitude. This NIH/University coop limits funding of 'small' projects and also Fogs the peer review process. (Is this sour grapes? Yep.) Is it that the reviewers are simply not qualified to pass quality scientific judgement on a manuscript? Or, to some extent is it politics in that the journals are remiss to print anything which might be looked on as a potential breakthrough and thereby adversely impact a significant group of investigators who regularly use their journal for turn the crank publications? Don't rock the boat? I don't know. While I am referencing many articles published in peer review journals, my personal experiences have been highly negative since I retired 20 years ago. Perhaps its jut me BUT, see chapter 18.

Chapter 18:   DRIVEL.

Drivel is the name for a new biomedical journal, which should be commissioned by Congress and published by the Library of Medicine. It would make available, hard copy and on line, articles submitted by those whose manuscripts have failed peer review or not sent for peer review. Authors would state and justify why their work deserves publication. Manuscripts would contain author names, title of article, abstract, key words, and body of the work, with references.

Pub Med would be directed to include Drivel in their abstracting/listing service. There would be publication charges of such a degree that Drivel might become the government's only profit center. A topic excluded from Drivel would be articles dealing with sex; were are already overloaded with Hollywood, TV, Internet, and newsstand junk. Drivel would serve to counter the hundreds of peer review journals which have a monopoly on readership and absolute power. There would be no academic restrictions; even scientific opinions of truck drivers might qualify for publication. The main reason for Drivel would be to balance the system, i.e. it would allow an alternate publishing venue and **D**oesn't **R**equire **I**nane **V**enal **E**xasperating **L**ackeys.

Chapter 19: Estimated Costs to Reach Yes/No Decisions on Value of Above

Chapter 2: The one dog pre-nitrogen washout protocol - S12,500

Chapter 3: The one dog heart attack 5 minute delay protocol - $12,500

If results are positive, 10 patient pilot study wherein nitrogen washout begins in ambulance and continues for 60-90 minutes after cath lab reperfusion. Added costs would be the heliox and its delivery system and tests to assess post recovery cardiac performance vs historical results. - $25,000

Chapter 6: Autism: 40 patient, one year clinical pilot study.

Initial and one year ONSD determinations. - $80,000

20 patients (half) placed on carbonic anhydrase inhibitor for one year monitored monthly.   - $20,000

One year Nuc. Med. cerebral blood flow determinations. - $40,000

Standard clinical evaluations, monthly and PRN - $40,000

Chapter 7: Alzheimer's disease: 300 patients.

Patients and protocols identical to those studies by Carmichael (chapter 7). Project assumes that the ONSD strudy suggested at the end of chapter 7 is conducted and demonstartes positive correlation of ICPs and T2 white matter levels.

Initial studies;

Magnetic resonance to assess normal/increased ICP pressure by ONSD. Also T2 weighted study of white matter to assess level of MRI-T2 white matter hyperintensity. A nuclear medicine study to assess total and regional brain blood flow.

Three groups:

Group 1: Dosed with increasing levels of acetazolamide to decrease production of CSF. WMH and ONSD detrminations conducted quarterly . ONSD targeted values are to approach ICPs of 10mmHg or less.

Group 2: Same as group 1 with the addition of heliox washout of nitrogen from the body for two hours every day. Same imaging

Groupt 3: Two hour daily washout of nitrogen. Same imaging as above..

At one year, repeat same imaging studies as initially.

 Cost estimate $3,000,000

Chapter 9: Nitrogen Gas as a chemotherapeutic agent. Identify suitable small animal model wherein tumors can be grown with a vascular supply that can be isolated and occluded. Est. - $1,000.00

Grow tumors in 12 animals to adequate size and then, occlude vascular supply in 6 of them for 3-5 minutes. Then infuse nitrogen saturated saline for 3-6 minutes. Into tumor mass. Observe growth/shrinking in all 12 animals for 1-2 weeks.

      Total Cost Est. - $10,000

Chapter 10: Solvents as therapeutic agents for HIV and E-Bola. Pilot test only on HIV and only with ethyl-ether. Find government sponsored labs conducting HIV research. Identify 6 animals with high HIV blood titer. Three groups of two. Animals anesthetized deeply with ether for one, three and six hours, all with body temperatures lowered to ~94 degrees F. Allow/force return of respiration and allow overnight recovery. Take blood samples daily for one week to see if there is any efficacy in reducing blood HIV titer.

   Est. total cost $2,000 per animal - $12,000

TOTAL COSTS—Guestimates

Chapter 2,3	cardiovascular	$50,000
Chapter 6	autism	$180,000
Chapter 7	Alzheimer's	$3,000,000
Chapter 9	nitrogen chemotherapy	$10,000
Chapter 10	solvents for in vivo viral delipdation	$12,000

AFTWORD:

Thanks for reading this rambling 'science' purge. I did not take the time to develop a very readable manuscript. Instead, my goal was to pursue simple concepts which might lead to novel therapies for complex disease conditions. I am convinced that some, if not all, of the pilot studies outlined in the chapters above deserve funding for feasibility studies. They do not entail the use of new drugs, nor the development of new equipment. Instead, they simply suggest new methods for use of existing drugs and technology. As a retired scientist, I can't conduct, manage or consult on any of these research efforts unless asked. I won't be.

There will be those who say: **This** can't be right because of that, that, that, that and that.

Well perhaps, much of **That** may be wrong because of this.

Folks: If you have loved ones suffering from any of the disease conditions considered in this book, you need to contact your state and federal government representatives and lobby for funding. With all the wasted BS spending in this country, the argument can't be - we don't have the money.

Disclaimers: Some of the thoughts and ideas may have been partially covered in other publications; that I acknowledge and herein credit. However, ideas, data and disclosure that appear herein which I believe to be novel are, that nitrogen gas is the cause of mitochondrial swelling, that the physiological function of the mitochondrial permeability transition pore is to function as an oxygen pump in a feedback loop, and that total body nitrogen washout may be of value in acute and chronic tissue hypoxia/anoxia. Also the observation of ONSD as an indicator of increased ICP in autism and the commentaries from chapters 9 through 11.

Donald R. VanDeripe, PhD

www.ingramcontent.com/pod-product-compliance
Lightning Source LLC
Chambersburg PA
CBHW080651180526
45168CB00008B/3386